Ultimate Paleo Diet For Beginners!

Paleo

Instant Paleo Weight Loss Tips And Recipes To Get In Shape, Lose Weight, Build Muscle, And Transform Your Body Fast!

I0417117

Sarah Brooks

STOP!!! Before you read any further....Would you like to know the Secrets of Body Transformation?

If your answer is yes, then you are not alone. Thousands of people are looking for the secret to rapidly burn body fat, keep the weight off, become healthier, and truly transform their body and life for good.

If you have been searching for these answers without much luck, you are in the right place!

Not only will you gain incredible insight in this book, but because I want to make sure to give you as much value as possible, right now for a limited time you can get full **100% FREE access to a VIP bonus EBook** entitled **THE 7 KEYS TO BODY TRANSFORMATION!**

Just Go Here For Free Instant Access:

www.liveFitVIP.com

Legal Notice

Disclaimer Notice

Table Of Contents

Introduction

I want to thank you and congratulate you for purchasing the book, *Paleo: Ultimate Paleo Diet For Beginners! Instant Paleo Weight Loss Tips And Recipes To Get In Shape, Lose Weight, Build Muscle, And Transform Your Body Fast!*

This book contains proven steps and strategies on how to lose weight effectively and keep your body strong and healthy. It is true that what we eat affects our overall health. Having said that, it is important that we know what we eat and consume only foods that are good for our body.

The Paleo diet allows you to eat all the foods that you want, without sacrificing taste and nutrition. Many people wonder how a caveman diet can be done during these modern times. It may not be easy at first, but this book will help you decide which foods are good for you and which are not.

In this book, you will:

- Learn how to choose foods that are Paleo-accepted.

- Know the benefits of Paleo diet and how it affects your health.

- Learn how to use Paleo effectively to build muscles and lose weight fast and effectively.

Although many diets are out there, the Paleo Diet has been proven effective by many and it has stood the tests of time. Even skeptics have seen the light and realized how beneficial the Paleo Diet is.

Thanks again for purchasing this book, I hope you enjoy it!

Chapter 1: Paleo Basics – What Does It Mean To Eat Paleo?

The Paleo Diet, short for Paleolithic Age Diet, aims to mimic the diet that our ancestors had long before agriculture came to the scene. During the Paleolithic era, our ancestors hunt their food, meaning they only eat free-range animals and any available fruits and vegetables in the wild. In our modern times, the Paleo diet means consuming grass-fed animals and organic fruits and vegetables. It's hard to replicate the caveman diet precisely; but the core idea is to eat unprocessed whole foods that contain all the proteins, nutrients and even the carbohydrates that our body needs.

Paleo diet means dumping the processed, refined, genetically-modified fruits, vegetables and meat and replacing them with farm-raised animals, fruits and vegetables. Note that most modern diseases such as autoimmune diseases, cancer and Type II Diabetes started to surface after industrialized foods or processed foods took upon the shelves of supermarkets and groceries.

Contrary to what many people know, finding the proper ingredients suitable for Paleo diet is not that hard. In fact, when you choose to go Paleo, you are actually helping small farmers make a better living. Paleo ingredients are often found in the farmer's markets. In general, small farmers grow their own fruits and vegetables in their small lands and usually use the traditional way of farming. Farm animals are also grown traditionally and are free from chemicals that are usually injected to commercial animals for them to be processed into foods at an earlier time.

Some farmers may use pesticides in their crops. This is something you should watch out for. Therefore, the best way to ensure that you are getting the best is to use organic foods. They are much more expensive, but the health and nutrition they provide is none compared to the money you spend. In case you can't get hold of organic foods, just make sure to stay away from any processed foods, sugar, legumes and grains that contain gluten.

Following the Paleo diet plan is not that hard. You don't even need to count your calories, nor do you need to give up your favorite foods. You just need to substitute unhealthy foods with whole unprocessed ones. The good news is that Paleo foods are tasty and packed with all the nutrients that you need.

Benefits of the Paleo diet

The following are some of the benefits that you will gain from sticking to a Paleo diet:

- Sustained weight loss

- Increased energy

- Increased muscle growth and fitness

- Reduced risk of diabetes, cancer and heart diseases

- Better nutrient absorption

- Higher immunity

- Improved glucose tolerance

- Healthy cells and brain

- Better digestion and gut health

- Reduced inflammation and allergies

- Increased sensitivity to insulin

- Reduced bloating

Chapter 2: Is Paleo Gluten-Free? How Does Eating Paleo Affect Your Blood Sugar

Gluten is a composite of two proteins: gliadin and glutenin that give dough its elastic texture. Gluten is commonly found in grains such as cereals, wheat, barley, rye and triticale. Gluten acts as the glue and keeps the food together to maintain their shape. People with celiac disease are sensitive to gluten. Gluten causes migraine, headaches, bloating, gas, diarrhea and vomiting as a result of celiac disease, which is an autoimmune disorder affecting the small intestine and the digestive process.

Paleo diet discourages the consumption of grains, starches and legumes, dairy, processed sugars, processed foods and alcohol. It also promotes the consumption of lean meats, fruits, vegetables, seafood, healthy fats, nuts and seeds. This means that the Paleo diet is gluten-free and is ideal for those who suffer from Celiac disease and Type II diabetes.

The Paleo diet concentrates on munching healthy fruits and vegetables, keeping away legumes, starches and grains. For some Paleo dieters, dairy is a no-no; but there are non-dairy alternatives if you wish to use one. Going Paleo does not mean you have to settle for tasteless, bland recipes. It's actually the other way around. With Paleo, you get to enjoy tasty, delicious dishes that are also very healthy and nutritious.

If you look closely, there is a great similarity between the Paleo diet and gluten-free diet. Perhaps the main difference is the motivation. For many, going Paleo means eliminating bad foods and consuming healthier, more nutritious foods for better health and well-being. Those who choose to follow the gluten-free diet usually do so for medical reasons. Celiac disease and gluten intolerance is gradually increasing. These medical conditions were once taught to be rare, but it has been proven otherwise. There are also those who switch to gluten-free diet because they think it is healthier.

How does eating Paleo affect your blood sugar?

Most diabetes sufferers wonder how the Paleo diet affects blood sugar and if this diet is good for them. Paleo diet is definitely ideal for Type 2 diabetes patients. This is because the Paleo diet does not include grains and refined sugars that cause the blood sugar to spike up. Instead, Paleo diet requires you to eat nutritious foods that provide a lot of benefits to your body.

A lot of people eat carbohydrate-rich foods. If you eat too much carbohydrates, then your body will be forced to store glucose in the fat cells instead of in your muscles; this will eventually cause insulin resistance. Glucose overload will also cause some glucose to enter your bloodstream; this leads to systemic inflammation that contributes to insulin resistance.

The Paleo diet normalizes your blood sugar level by ensuring that you follow a diet and lifestyle which prevents the unhealthy spike of your blood sugar level. Since the Paleo diet requires you to stay away from carbohydrates, you no longer need to worry about huge glucose spikes that will eventually lead to insulin resistance.

The diet plan also requires you to stay away from processed foods that can trigger autoimmune responses. It prevents you from getting overly exposed to toxins. Since the Paleo diet is also free of lectins and gluten that cause leaky gut or systemic inflammation, you have a guarantee that your blood sugar level won't immediately spike up. Most of those who undergo the Paleo diet also say that they were able to normalize their blood sugar levels within just a short period of time.

Chapter 3: The Proper Way To Eat Paleo For Building More Muscles

Aside from all the health benefits that this diet offers, Paleo diet can also help you build some muscles. The diet plan requires you to live and eat healthy, which is a huge help when trying to achieve a better physique. There might be a few tweaks here and there but nonetheless, it's still healthy and will definitely give you a healthier, leaner and stronger physique.

Going Paleo means there is no need to monitor your caloric intake since the ingredients are whole, unprocessed foods anyways; but if you are trying to build some muscle mass, sticking to a strict low-carb Paleo diet may not suit your needs. You will definitely get leaner with Paleo but if you want more muscles, you need carbohydrates. To build more muscles, you can have organic potatoes, sweet potatoes and white rice as your main sources of carbohydrates.

Doing this will allow you to get your needed calories while still staying away from refined sugars and gluten-rich grains such as cereals, wheat, rye and barley. When trying to build muscles using the Paleo diet, you are not allowed to consume cereal bars, sugar-filled soda and artificial sauces as well as candy bars. You have to stick to the all-natural sources only.

To make it easier for you, just follow the list below.

Foods to be taken to build more muscle mass:

- Grass-fed red meat
- Lean poultry meat (breast)
- Fish (All types)
- Free range eggs
- Organic whole dairy products
- Whey protein

Foods that can be consumed to build more muscles, but in moderation:

- Poultry meat (leg and skin) can be consumed 1 to 2 times a week

- Raw nuts

- Fried foods (in olive oil only, no vegetable oil or other processed oils)

- Raw honey

- Sugary fruits such as cherry, banana, pineapples and the likes

Foods to be avoided at any cost if you want to build muscles while on a Paleo diet:

- Any processed foods

- All processed meats

- Skimmed dairy products

- Foods with Omega 6 (Polyunsaturated) – vegetable oils, vegetable spreads, deep-fried foods, mayonnaise and roasted, salted, honey roasted nuts

- Refined carbohydrates and grains or foods with refined sugar and high gluten content – sugar, cereals, soda, cakes, pastries, biscuits, cookies, etc.

To build muscles while you are on a Paleo diet, you need to eat foods that are rich in protein and eliminate sugars and gluten. You can start seeing a noticeable increase in your muscle mass and strength within just three months of sticking to the Paleo diet plan.

Chapter 4: The Best Way To Eat Paleo For Fat Loss

Some dieters tend to lose hope and become frustrated if they don't see their desired weight loss results after exerting a lot of effort. There are those who lose weight at the start and tend to gain this back after returning to their old habits. This is not the case when you decide to stick to the Paleo diet plan. This is because you won't feel deprived. You can still eat the foods that you want. Paleo allows you to stick to a diet plan which is suitable enough for your body. With Paleo, you can eat some of the foods that you are craving for; but you need to choose the ingredients well.

Take for example some sweet delights such as cakes. You are still allowed to eat cakes, but you need to look for substitutes for unhealthy ingredients that may only ruin your fat loss efforts. Instead of using wheat flour or all purpose flour, you can use almond flour, coconut flour or arrowroot flour instead. These are gluten-free substitutes and they taste great. At first, you may feel that something is missing with the taste since your body is used to sugar and other preservatives; but, with just a few adjustments to the ingredients, it is not hard to come along.

You have to understand that gaining weight is not all about eating too much of everything. Your lifestyle is also a big part of the equation. Just like any other diet, you also need to move, drink enough water and have enough sleep to ensure a healthier body. Staying away from bad vices such as smoking and alcohol is also a must.

To make it simple, Paleo means to cut off bad, processed foods and keep your body moving while getting enough sleep. Below is a method you can follow for an effective Paleo weight loss. This is after you have thrown all processed foods you can find in your house, started walking a bit and tried getting enough sleep for a day.

- Reduce your consumption of starchy carbohydrates and fruits. Your goal is to get the majority of your carbohydrates from fibrous fruits and vegetables. Eat more red meat, such as beef or bison or any other pastured red meat that are grass-fed since they are calorie dense.

- Start having a regular physical routine such as walking every morning for 30 minutes. After a month, you can increase your physical activity. You may start lifting light weights, go swimming, surfing or any activity of your choice on a regular interval. Pair your physical activities with a healthy Paleo diet and you will be on your way towards losing a lot of fat.

- After the first month, there should be no more gluten-rich grains on your diet. Wheat, barley, rye and cereals should be eliminated. Dairy products and refined sugars should also be eliminated. Here are the list of Paleo substitutes that you can use:

    - Free-range meat, free-range poultry or grass-fed and wild-caught fish

    - Free-range eggs

    - Non-dairy milk such as coconut milk and almond milk

    - Non-dairy whipped cream or coconut cream

    - Raw nuts only. Peanuts are legumes so they should be eliminated.

    - Non-dairy ice cream such as coconut ice cream.

    - Almond flour/meal, coconut flour or arrowroot flour in place of wheat flour or all-purpose flour

    - Non-refined coconut oil for cooking

    - Avocado oil and virgin coconut oil for salads.

    - Cassava or tapioca starch in place of cornstarch

    - Organic cacao powder or butter as substitute for chocolate

- Raw honey or coconut crystals. Avoid using mesquite honey or clover honey as these are legumes. As a precaution, honey should not be fed to children 1 year old and under as it may pose health hazards.

- Unfiltered apple cider vinegar to replace all types of vinegar

- Use sea salt or pink Himalayan salt sparingly

Avoid using canned fruits or spices as much as possible. It is best to use fresh vegetables, fruits and spices. You may find Paleo dishes difficult to achieve but it all depends on you. Keep your dishes simple by using simple ingredients. For example, you can cook delicious omelet for breakfast by just beating up some free-range eggs, a pinch of sea salt and some chopped fresh basil.

For lunch, you can have roasted fish with some fresh fruits for side dish and a glass of orange juice. You can also find easy-to-bake Paleo cakes and pastries online if you crave for something sweet.

Chapter 5: Sample Workout Routine For Building Muscle

To build muscles effectively using the Paleo diet, you should have a workout routine. Remember to eat enough prior to and after your workout. Avoid depriving yourself of food since this might only cause you to overeat in the long run. Since your goal for working out is to build more muscles, it is advisable to supply your body with enough carbohydrates. Just make sure that you get your daily dose of carbohydrates from healthy food sources that won't ruin your Paleo meal plans. A few good sources are sweet potatoes and red lean meat.

This chapter focuses on discussing a few workout routines that you can pair with your Paleo diet to boost your chances of building lean muscles. Consider doing the workouts mentioned in this chapter early in the morning after drinking a glass of freshly squeezed orange juice. It is also crucial for you to target your upper body (back, chest, triceps, biceps and shoulder muscles) and your lower body (hamstrings, abs, calves and quads) to ensure getting the best results out of your muscle building workout routines.

Best Upper Body Workout Routines

These upper body workout routines should be done at least 2 to 3 times per week.

Bench Press – Do three sets consisting of six to eight repetitions. Take a 2 to 3-minute rest in between sets.

Incline Dumbbell Press – Do three sets consisting of eight to ten repetitions. A 1 to 2-minute rest in between sets is highly recommended.

Lat Pull-downs - Do three sets with eight to ten repetitions. It is also advisable to have one to two minutes of rest.

Lateral Raises – Do two sets with ten to twelve repetitions. 1-minute rest would suffice.

Dumbbell Curls – Do two sets with ten to twelve repetitions. You can also take a 1-minute rest after each set.

Best Lower Body Workout Routines

These lower body workout routines should also be performed 2 to 3 times weekly.

Pull-ups – It is highly recommended to have three sets with six to eight repetitions and 2 to 3-minute rests.

Seated Cable Row – Do three sets composed of eight to ten repetitions. Rest for one to two minutes after each set.

Dumbbell Flyes – Do two sets with ten to twelve repetitions. A 1-minute rest is highly recommended.

Skull Crushers – Do two sets of the skull crushers workout routine with ten to twelve repetitions each. You can take a 1-minute break after each set.

Barbell Curls – Perform two sets with ten to twelve reps.

You can have alternating workout routines; this means that you can do the upper body workout on Monday, lower body workout on Tuesday, upper body workout on Wednesday, and so on. This will give the muscles in both body parts time to recover from the strenuous exercise. It is important that you follow your Paleo diet while you are doing these routines.

You may follow the diet for building lean muscles discussed on the earlier chapter to ensure that you will achieve a stronger body with lean muscles faster. Do not use any sugar-filled products. Increase your consumption of red lean meat and stay away from alcohol and smoking. It is also important to eat 5 to 6 meals a day to help you gain more muscle mass faster.

Chapter 6: Sample Workout Routine For Shredding Body Fat

Losing body fat is not an easy journey but it is achievable. You just need to be consistent with your exercise routines and stick to your Paleo diet. Remember that enough sleep is also important if you really want to shed those extra pounds.

Full Body Workout

- 5 reps (10 RM) for each exercise

- Conventional Deadlift for 6 minutes

- Chest Supported Dumbbell Row for 6 minutes

- Bulgarian Split Squat for 6 minutes

- Barbell Complex 3 x 6 exercise (bent over row, back squat and hang power clean to push press)

- 100 Inverted suspension row (as fast as you can)

Follow this workout routine consistently. Consider Saturdays and Sundays as your days off from exercise to give your muscles and some of your body parts enough time to recover. Increase the number of minutes by 2 minutes each day for conventional deadlift, chest supported dumbbell row and Bulgarian split squat.

The barbell complex and inverted suspension row should be done consistently for the entire week. For the next coming weeks, you can add 5 to 10 lbs to the weight that you used the week before.

Remember to eat as needed since this will serve as your fuel to do your workout. Do not starve yourself as this will impede your weight loss. Stick to your all-natural Paleo diet and the exercise routine mentioned in this chapter and you will start noticing a huge difference in your weight in just a week.

Chapter 7: Tips For Building Muscle And Losing Fat To Transform Your Body As Fast As Possible

To ensure that you build lean muscles and lose your body fast faster while you are on a Paleo diet, follow these simple tips:

- Drink lots of water. To calculate the amount of water you need to consume in one day, get your body weight in pounds and divide it by two. Change the pounds into ounces and convert this to liters. For example, if you weigh 250 lbs., you should divide that figure by two; the result is 125 oz. When you convert 125 oz. to liters, you will get 3.7 liters or roughly 4 liters. Therefore, you need to drink 4 liters of water in a day.

- Get enough sleep. Studies have shown that lack of sleep affects body fats. If you want to see significant changes in your body faster, you should make an effort to achieve at least 6 to 8 hours of sleep in a day. You can sleep from 8pm to 4am, 9pm to 5am or anywhere near those times.

- Eat more with smaller servings. When you feel hungry, eat. Do not starve yourself. Starvation harms the body and impedes healthy weight loss. Eat but do not overeat. Instead of having 3 large meals in a day, divide it to 5 or 6 smaller portions. Since you are building lean muscles, add more red meat and lean poultry meat to your diet.

- Do not eliminate carbohydrates from your diet. You need carbohydrates for energy. Since you are doing Paleo Diet and you are trying to build lean muscles, sweet potatoes and rice are good sources of carbohydrates; but you have to consume them in moderation.

- Do not sleep right away after eating dinner. It is best to eat dinner an hour before going to bed. You have to give your body enough time to process the foods that you consumed before you go to sleep at night.

- Do not skip breakfast. Breakfast is the most important meal for the day since it helps your body sustain your energy level. Your breakfast should contain protein and carbohydrates.

- Add more green leafy vegetables to your diet. They are rich in fiber that helps in better digestion. Better digestion means that the nutrients from the foods you eat are absorbed effectively by your body. Furthermore, green, leafy vegetables also contain iron which is good for your red blood cells. These red blood cells are responsible for transporting nutrients all over your body.

Deciding to live healthy comes with a huge responsibility. You should stay away from "bad foods" and be consistent with your diet and exercise routines. Follow these simple tips and you will see great results immediately.

Chapter 8: Incredibly Delicious Paleo Diet Recipes To Get In Shape Fast And Love Eating Paleo

Eating Paleo should not put a toll on you. Although it may seem overwhelming at first, once you understand fully how the Paleo Diet works, everything will go smoothly. Here are easy to prepare Paleo dishes that are unbelievably delicious and nutritious. They are also very easy to prepare so you won't have to spend a lot of time in the kitchen.

Beef Zucchini Pasta

Ingredients:

800 grams minced grass-fed beef

¼ cup red pesto (without the cheese)

1 tbsp ghee or grass-fed butter

Fresh parsley

Pinch of sea salt or Pink Himalayan salt

800 lbs (about 4 medium) Zucchini noodles (shaped using a spiralizer or a julienne peeler)

Instructions:

If you are using frozen meat, thaw in advance to allow gradual defrosting. Heat a saucepan in medium heat and grease it with ghee or grass-fed butter. Place the meat and stir until it turns brown. Set the stove in low heat and add freshly chopped parsley and red pesto. Keep stirring. Turn off the heat and transfer the meat into a bowl. Remove the soft core of the zucchini and place in the spiralizer to make noodles.

If you are using a julienne peeler, keep peeling the zucchini around and stop when you reach the soft center. In the same saucepan, place the remaining ghee or grass-fed butter and stir in the zucchini noodles. Cook until tender. Add this to the meat and turn off the heat. Serve while hot.

Paleo Avocado Slaw

2 large avocados

¼ cup rice vinegar or apple cider vinegar

¼ coconut milk (full fat)

2 garlic cloves

1 tablespoon Dijon mustard

4 cups shredded cabbage

2 cups packaged broccoli slaw

½ teaspoon pepper

A pinch of sea salt or Himalayan pink salt

Instructions:

In a food processor, combine the avocado, meat, garlic, mustard, pepper and salt. Blend until mashed. Combine vinegar and slowly add coconut milk. Blend until smooth. In a large salad bowl, mix the broccoli, cabbage and avocado mixture. Mix until all vegetables are coated. You may serve right away or chill before serving.

Coco Lime Sweet Balls

Ingredients:

½ cup cashews

½ cup almonds

½ cup dates (pitted)

½ cup desiccated coconut (unsweetened)

3 key lime fruits (for juice and for zest)

Instructions:

In a food processor, pulse cashew and almonds until they are finely chopped. Add the pitted dates, lime zest and lime juice. Blend until dates are chopped finely and the mixture starts to clump. Get 1 tablespoonful of the mixture and shape into balls. Roll in coconut until the outer part is completely covered. Use an airtight container for storage and keep in the refrigerator. You can serve this for snacks or for dessert.

Sweet Potato Bacon Wraps

Ingredients:

9 to 10 slices nitrate-free or free-range bacon

2 medium sweet potatoes or yams (whichever is available)

Instructions:

Preheat oven to 400°F. Cut the sweet potatoes or yams into lengthwise wedges. Cut the bacon slices into two lengthwise pieces. Thinner bacon slices work better for this recipe.

Wrap each sweet potato or yam wedges with the bacon sliced lengthwise. You can stick the ends with a toothpick to prevent the bacon from separating while baking.

Line the sweet potato wraps in a rimmed baking sheet. Bake for 10 minutes and flip. Continue baking until the bacon strips are crispy. Serve immediately and enjoy!

Berry Vanilla Pudding

Ingredients:

400 ml coconut milk (full fat)

5 tablespoons Chia seeds

½ teaspoon vanilla extract

1 teaspoon Maca powder

½ cup raw honey

1 ½ cup fresh raspberries

1 ½ cup fresh blueberries

Instructions:

In a mixing bowl, combine the coconut milk, chia seeds, vanilla extract, raw honey and maca powder. Whisk until the mixture is no longer lumpy and the chia seeds are distributed evenly. Refrigerate and stir from time to time until the pudding becomes thick. It takes about an hour. If the pudding still has a thin texture, add one more tablespoon of chia seeds.

You may serve this pudding in serving cups or small mugs. Scoop a spoonful of pudding and layer it at the bottom of the mug. Top with blueberries and scoop another pudding and layer on top. Add raspberries. You can serve it the way you want. Just be creative about it. You may serve it immediately or keep in a tightly sealed container and refrigerate for later use.

Note: You may use strawberries instead. If available, you can sprinkle with ground almonds.

Spicy Chicken Wings

Ingredients:

1000 grams free-range chicken wings

1 lime (juiced)

2 Jalapeño peppers (seeds removed and cut into chunks)

4 cloves garlic, peeled

½ cup fresh cilantro leaves

1 teaspoon ground cumin

¼ cup coconut oil

2 tablespoons coconut aminos

Instructions:

Put all the ingredients in a blender (except for the chicken) and process until smooth. In a large tightly sealed container or a large freezer bag, pour the marinade and put the chicken wings inside. Toss the chicken wings until they are all evenly coated. Marinate overnight.

Preheat your oven to 200°C. Line your baking tray with foil and place a cooling rack on it. Line the chicken wings properly on the cooling rack. Bake for 15 minutes. Turn the chicken wings on the other side and bake for another 15 minutes or until the chicken wings turn brown.

Serve with Nuts and Spices dressing dip.

Ingredients:

¼ cup raw cashews (unsalted) – soak for 6 hours, rinse and drain

Half lemon (juiced)

½ cup coconut milk

1 tablespoon fresh chives, chopped

¼ teaspoon coarsely ground black pepper

½ teaspoon dried dill

½ teaspoon onion powder

½ teaspoon garlic powder

Pinch of sea salt

Instructions:

Blend or process the soaked and drained cashews until you reach the consistency of a paste. Scrape down the sides of your blender as necessary. Once the blended cashews reach a texture similar to a paste, you can add the coconut milk slowly until the mixture becomes smooth. Add the lemon juice and the herbs and continue blending. If it becomes too thick, add some water and reprocess.

Use this dip to enjoy your Spicy Chicken Wings even more.

Easy Bacon and Mushroom Casserole

Ingredients

2.5 lbs smoked, nitrate-free bacon

3 stems fresh spinach (stems removed)

1 lb sliced button mushrooms

1 large onions, chopped

2 garlic cloves, minced

2 tablespoons ghee or grass-fed butter

Some ground pepper

Sea salt to taste

Ingredients:

Cut the bacon into medium strips. Place the bacon strips in a non-stick pan and cook until oil comes out of the bacon. Make sure the bacon is soft and not crunchy. Add the onions and cook until soft. Toss in the minced garlic and continue cooking until fragrant.

Add mushrooms and stir. Cook for another 8 minutes or until mushrooms are soft. Add the butter or ghee and the spinach. Stir occasionally and turn off the heat when the spinach is already cooked. Season with ground pepper and some sea salt to taste. Serve.

Vegetable Sauté with Beef Strips

1 lb lean beef meat (cut thinly into strips)

1 small red onion, julienned

2 cloves garlic, crushed and minced

1 small red bell pepper, julienned

Ground black pepper

Sea salt

2 tablespoons coconut oil

1 small head cabbage (cut into long strips)

1 medium carrots (shaped into flowers or cut into thin strips)

A few onion leeks for toppings (chopped)

A cup of water

Instructions:

Add coconut oil into a pan and heat it using medium heat setting. Sauté the onion, garlic, red bell pepper and beef strips. When the beef is no longer red or when the color has turned to dark brown, add the carrots. Cook for a minute, stir and add the cabbage strips. Cook for another minute. Add water gradually until most of the vegetables are covered. Sprinkle with salt and pepper to taste. Remove from heat and top with chopped onion leeks. Serve with brown rice while hot.

Breakfast Protein Pancake

Ingredients

2 large bananas (mashed)

2 large eggs (whisked)

½ cup vanilla protein powder

Non-dairy chocolate chips (this is optional; you may substitute it with dried fruits if you prefer)

1 tablespoon butter or oil for greasing the pan

Instructions:

Mix the mashed bananas, eggs and vanilla protein powder in a bowl until well-blended. Heat the pan over medium heat and grease with butter or oil. When the pan is hot enough, add about 3 to 5 inches wide of the pancake mixture.

Sprinkle some chocolate chips or dried fruits on top. Once the sides start to bubble, turn the pancake over and cook the other side. Cook for about a minute or until brown. Redo the process and grease the pan when needed.

This recipe is ideal for people on the go since it only takes a few minutes to prepare.

Conclusion

Thank you again for purchasing this book on how to lose weight effectively with Paleo Diet!

I am extremely excited to pass this information along to you, and I am so happy that you now have read and can hopefully implement these strategies going forward.

I hope this book was able to help you understand clearly what a Paleo diet is and how to use it to obtain leaner muscles, increase your strength and have a healthier body. It is not too late to be healthy and get the body you always wanted. Paleo Diet is extremely effective if done properly and this is what this book is all about – to help you understand Paleo and be able to use it so that you can have a healthier, stronger and leaner body for a better life experience.

The next step is to get started using this information and to hopefully live a healthy and worry-free life!

Please don't be someone who just reads this information and doesn't apply it, the strategies in this book will only benefit you if you use them!

If you know of anyone else that could benefit from the information presented here please inform them of this book.

Finally, if you enjoyed this book and feel it has added value to your life in any way, please take the time to share your thoughts and post a review on Amazon. It'd be greatly appreciated!

Thank you and good luck!

Preview Of:

Ultimate Coconut Oil Guide!

<u>Coconut Oil</u>

Coconut Oil Recipes For Organic Skin Care And Natural Beauty, Clean Eating For Weight Loss, Shinning Hair, Better Brain Function And Overall Health!

Table Of Contents

Introduction

I want to thank you and congratulate you for purchasing the book, *Coconut Oil: Ultimate Coconut Oil Guide! - Coconut Oil Recipes For Organic Skin Care And Natural Beauty, Clean Eating For Weight Loss, Shining Hair, Better Brain Function And Overall Health!*

This book contains proven steps and strategies on how you can take full advantage of the beauty, weight loss and health benefits that coconut oil has to offer. Through this book, you will learn more about:

- What makes coconut oil healthy?

- How it can help you get better, more glowing skin.

- Its effects on your hair and making healthier.

- Can coconut oil improve your brain function?

- Weight loss benefits and how it can boost your metabolism.

- Coconut oil and how it can help treat different illnesses.

- Recipes for both your diet as well as organic skin care.

- How to choose the right coconut oil for your needs.

We hope that through this book, you'll be able to recognize the amount of potential that a single bottle of coconut oil contains.

Thanks again for purchasing this book, I hope you enjoy it!

Chapter 1: Coconut Oil For Natural Beauty And Health

These days, more and more people are becoming aware of the effects that chemically manufactured products has on their bodies. As such, many of them have turned to a greener, more organic lifestyle that advocates going all natural when it comes to their food as well as the different products that they use on their bodies.

This isn't surprising, of course, considering the fact that there are a number of illnesses which are associated with constant use of synthetic and often chemical-laden skin and health products. There are certain risks that one must bear when using it; risks which can be avoided altogether if one were to switch over to something that's a bit closer to nature.

The coconut oil is a favorite among health buffs as it is one of those by-products that can be used in a multitude of ways. On one hand, it can be eaten and taken as a supplement which would boost your overall health. On the other, it can be applied topically and used as a beauty product as well as a means of treating certain skin issues.

You get all of these benefits but without worrying about its harmful effects to the body.

Why is it considered one of the best natural remedies out there?

It's all in the composition. About 99% of it is composed of saturated fats (which, in this case isn't as bad as it sounds) as well as traces of polyunsaturated fatty acids and monosaturated fatty acids. Virgin coconut oil retains a higher amount of the good stuff thus it is also valued higher.

It also contains lauric acid and quite a generous amount of it at that. When digested by the body, this would turn into monolaurin and is very beneficial when it comes to dealing with different bacteria and viruses. Diseases such as influenza and herpes are just two of the things that coconut oil can cure in a jiff. A tablespoon of it a day keeps the doctor away, so to speak.

Besides these, it is also one of the most powerful inhibitors of quite a number of different pathogenic organisms ranging from your usual viruses to even protozoa. All of this, of course, is attributed to its high lauric acid content.

For beauty and skincare

Coconut can also be used for cosmetic or skin care purposes. We'll get to the specifics of this in later chapters but to quickly summarize, it is often used for: Hair care, skin care, nails, lips as well as treating different skin issues such as psoriasis. It helps keep the skin youthful and glowing as well as protect it from harmful UV rays.

Thanks for Previewing My Exciting Book

"Coconut Oil: Ultimate Coconut Oil Guide! Coconut Oil Recipes For Organic Skin Care And Natural Beauty, Clean Eating For Weight Loss, Shinning Hair, Better Brain Function And Overall Health!"

To purchase this book, simply go to the Amazon Kindle store and simply search:

"COCONUT OIL"

Then just scroll down until you see my book. You will know it is mine because you will see my name "Sarah Brooks" underneath the title.

Alternatively, you can visit my author page on Amazon to see this book and other work I have done. Thanks so much, and please don't forget your free bonuses

DON'T LEAVE YET! - CHECK OUT YOUR FREE BONUSES BELOW!

Free Bonus Offer: Get Free Access To The www.LiveFitVIP.com VIP Newsletter!

Once you enter your email address you will immediately get free access to this awesome newsletter!

But wait, right now if you join now for free you will also get free access to the "The 7 Keys To Body Transformation" free EBook!

To claim both your FREE VIP NEWSLETTER MEMBERSHIP and your FREE BONUS eBook on THE 7 KEYS TO BODY TRANSFORMATION!

Just Go To:

www.liveFitVIP.com

www.ingramcontent.com/pod-product-compliance
Lightning Source LLC
Chambersburg PA
CBHW070937290526
45795CB00003B/1051